T0067127

My Kid's a Picky Eater

*Twelve Secrets to Changing
Your Child's Eating Habits*

Laura Kopec

BALBOA
PRESS

A DIVISION OF HAY HOUSE

Balboa Press books may be ordered through booksellers or by contacting:

Balboa Press
A Division of Hay House
1663 Liberty Drive
Bloomington, IN 47403
www.balboapress.com
1 (877) 407-4847

Because of the dynamic nature of the Internet, any web addresses or links contained in this book may have changed since publication and may no longer be valid. The views expressed in this work are solely those of the author and do not necessarily reflect the views of the publisher, and the publisher hereby disclaims any responsibility for them.

The author of this book does not dispense medical advice or prescribe the use of any technique as a form of treatment for physical, emotional, or medical problems without the advice of a physician, either directly or indirectly. The intent of the author is only to offer information of a general nature to help you in your quest for emotional and spiritual well-being. In the event you use any of the information in this book for yourself, which is your constitutional right, the author and the publisher assume no responsibility for your actions.

Any people depicted in stock imagery provided by Thinkstock are models, and such images are being used for illustrative purposes only.
Certain stock imagery © Thinkstock.

Printed in the United States of America.

ISBN: 978-1-5043-2656-8 (sc)
ISBN: 978-1-5043-2657-5 (e)

Library of Congress Control Number: 2015900623

Balboa Press rev. date: 02/10/2015

To Eden, Luke and Sierra
Thank you for all you have taught me.
I love you, Mom

CONTENTS

FOREWORD

My name is Holly Willis and I am a certified and licensed pediatric speech language pathologist. While I work with a variety of disorders, I specialize in feeding disorders. I have worked closely with Laura Kopec for a number of years, personally and professionally. She has not only improved the quality of my life with nutritional counseling, but also the lives of many others. I have been impressed with her background, knowledge, and flexibility to meet people where they are in their journey to improved health.

I am also a mother of a child who has always been a bit of a picky eater. So, I can't tell you how eager I was to read *My Kid's a Picky Eater*. I was looking forward to some great ideas for parents like me, and I was not disappointed. This book is loaded with helpful information to encourage parents and motivate children of all ages to break out of their poor eating habits in a very positive way.

It is one thing to know that your child is not eating enough of a variety that would be considered a well-balanced diet. It is an entirely different beast to know what to do about it. For many parents, it is easier to take the road of least resistance and just give them what you know they will eat. It may be chicken nuggets at every meal, but they have to eat something or they'll starve, right? Then what do you do when they get sick of eating that one food item because that's all they will eat? Laura clearly understands that we as parents can't simply reason with our children and tell them what is good for them and they will just eat it because we said so. I wish it was that easy, but unfortunately it is not. Those little people have minds of their own!

While Laura does not claim to have the cure for picky eating, she has given the reader a great place to start their journey in an attempt to increase their child's willingness to try new foods. A well-balanced diet with a variety of foods is extremely important for your child's overall cognitive, physical and emotional development. Let this book assist you in helping your child become a better version of themselves.

Holly Willis, M.S., CCC-SLP

ACKNOWLEDGEMENTS

I would like to thank each and every Mom that has come into my office on behalf of their picky eater. You are courageous and commendable. May you continue to prioritize the health and well-being of your children. Thank you for the inspiration to reach other Moms by writing this book.

I am grateful to my editor, Anita Battista for her candor and strong commitment to her work. I am blessed to know you.

I would like to thank the many health care professionals that have recommended me and my work to many mothers with nutritional questions. Thank you for your trust and recognition.

I am thankful to my husband, Anthony Orchard and his dedication to our family and his efforts in our financial well being.

I would like to thank Holly Willis, MS, CCC-SLP for her feedback, comments and her wonderful contribution to this book.

I am grateful to Liza Orchard for her creative genius and her artistry. I love her work and her wit. Her book cover designs are brilliant.

I would like to thank my dear friend and soul-sister Beverly Wells. She knows all the reasons why.

I am blessed for my precious family that is so very valuable to me especially the support of Dan Kopec, Jerry Kopec, Marc Cook, Pat Loewy, John and Diane Kopec, and Kevin Kopec.

I am thankful to my girlfriends Kari Berry and Alex Hyman who believe in me and inspire me to keep going no matter what.

I would like to thank Sherry Wiggins, Samantha Naidoo, Karin Proctor, and Amanda Orchard Fernandez who contributed in some way to the creation of this book.

A special thank you to Jonie Slater, MS, OTR/L for her contributions, expertise and feedback.

I would like to thank my loyal and hard working assistant, Karimen Montero. I wish her luck in all her endeavors.

I am grateful to the child rearing experts whose books I devour, that I hope one day to meet, Dr. Kevin Leman and Madeline Levine who have greatly influenced how I have grown as a parent.

A NOTE TO THE READER

The information in this book is provided to educate the reader. Any decision involving the treatment of an illness or condition should be made only after consulting a physician or health care practitioner of your choice. Neither this nor any book can guarantee complete absence of disease nor substitute professional medical care or treatment. The information contained in this book is not intended to serve as a replacement for professional medical advice. Any use of the information in this book is at the reader's discretion. The author and the publisher specifically disclaim any and all liability arising directly or indirectly from the use or application of any information contained in this book. A health care professional should be consulted regarding your specific situation. The client names have been eliminated in specific stories to protect their privacy.

INTRODUCTION

In my consulting practice I see many faces. Many of those faces are loving and hardworking moms who want the very best for their children. These moms wish their children would eat better and eat healthier but these moms have no idea how to begin to make these changes. They call their child a "picky eater." Many of these moms were frustrated and felt their picky eater was a lost battle. Many of these moms felt desperate to change their picky eater.

Each of these moms came into my office hoping that I would present a solution for resolving the picky eater believing the blame was in food. They were hoping they had missed some magic recipe for getting their child to eat vegetables. Many thought there might be a smoothie their child would love and make the picky eater problem disappear. Many were really surprised to find out there is no recipe per say, but a different style of understanding nutrition and behavior and putting the new understanding and behavior into place.

Maybe this sounds like you. Maybe you have one: the child who won't eat their vegetables, or won't eat a meal without a favorite video playing, the child who only wants sugar treats or "bad carbs" or maybe you just have a feeling your child does not eat as well as they should.

The picky eater can have one or more characteristics that ultimately keep him or her from eating healthy foods on a continual basis.

Through the years I have had the opportunity to meet with so many moms and create nutritional plans for the picky eater that includes some of the very information contained in this book. More and more moms come back in only two to four weeks and report positive changes happening not only for their picky eater, but also their entire family as well. They realize good nutrition for their child began with their understanding as a parent and the strategies they implemented from there.

I wrote this book for parents struggling with a typical picky eater. But I want to be clear, while this book is for every parent, it may not help every child. This book contains important information for every parent and every family, but some of the information may or may not specifically help all aspects of your child's issues if your child's eating habits make your child a *problem feeder* which is different from a *picky eater.*

All the information in this book may not apply if your child's eating behavior has to do with a sensory disorder, a GI tube, dysphagia (swallowing difficulties), oral motor impairments (including low tone and poor coordination), sensory aversions to foods based on smell, appearance and texture, or sensory issues associated with the Autism Spectrum Disorder. If your child is dealing with one or more of the issues stated above you may need a speech pathologist or occupational therapist who is experienced with feeding disorders to help you determine if your child has a motor, sensory or structural behavioral cause related to medical issues leading to feeding difficulties. There are many professionals in this arena to help you determine the difference between a picky eater and a problem feeder.

If your child's issues are related to digestive imbalances you may need personal nutritional counseling that either includes a digestive assessment and or comprehensive digestive testing in addition to the strategies in this book. There is tremendous value in establishing the health of your child's digestive system with the information I provide through nutritional counseling.

Regardless of your child's condition, I believe all children can still benefit from the information contained in this book. I hope you find relevant and important information for you and your whole family. I hope this book presents many possible solutions for your picky eater before the habits are permanent and the health costs great. Take each chapter slowly and make changes at your own pace. Use the end of each chapter's *Tips and Summary* as a helpful guide. Most of all remember your entire family can benefit from eating more healthy foods and being healthy eaters.

SECRET #1

Understand the Problem

We want the best for our children. We want to be really good parents. Yet, we often feel judged by how many activities our children are involved in, how well they are excelling at one or more of these activities, or how much technology they have or what kind of phone they use. As a result, we have pushed our children, stressed them, overextended them, and in the end, may very well have done more harm than good. Leading experts in today's child psychology speak to us about the dangers of over scheduling and over extending our children and the cost to their mental and emotional well-being. As a result, we may be missing some basics. What if we found out that two of the most important factors influencing a child's wellbeing and success are time together as a family, especially mealtimes, and nutrition? How would we change what we are doing? Might we take a hard look at what we think matters in the life of our child, where our focus should be, and what priorities might come first?

A typical child's diet contains almost no fruits and vegetables.[1] Most children are eating the bulk of their calories from white flour, sugar, oil, and dairy. The consequences of a diet primarily consisting of these kinds of refined foods containing white flour, sugar, and oil may lead to serious illness and disease such as cancer and autoimmune disease.[2] We now know that many diseases are often preventable with changes in diet and lifestyle. The American Cancer Society even suggests eating two and a half cups of fruit and vegetables as one of its diet and lifestyle recommendations for preventing cancer.[3] Of course, the earlier you begin healthy habits the easier it is to be consistent. It stands to reason if healthy eating is a learned behavior, the food choices our children are making now may influence their physical, mental and emotional health for years to come. As parents, we may have a greater chance of influencing the diet and lifestyle factors that affect physical, mental, and emotional health if we understand them and take action.

The simple fact is we are machines that run on a certain kind of fuel—natural and wholesome foods. We can get by on inadequate fuels but eventually we will pay the consequences of eating poorly. Natural and whole foods are the raw materials that our cells need to be nourished. Natural and whole foods make up the macronutrients of protein, good carbohydrates and healthy fats that give us energy, brain power and physical benefits such as muscle tone. Within those macronutrients are micronutrients – the vitamins and minerals that provide vital nutrition for all the inner and outer workings of our bodies. For example, we know that Beta Carotene is important for eye health. This great micronutrient is often found in the macronutrient carbohydrate known as carrots.

Unfortunately, very few children eat carrots on a regular basis. Very few children eat carrots, broccoli, spinach, kale, cabbage and apples on a regular basis. If your child eats a diet consisting mainly refined carbohydrates or sugar foods then they may be on a destructive path where their academic, athletic and interpersonal performance may be affected by long term consequences of chronic conditions such as ulcerative colitis or acid reflux, to heart disease, diabetes, obesity and cancer. You may feel overwhelmed by the inability to influence his or her eating. You may feel like they will only eat macaroni and cheese or nothing, or chicken nuggets or nothing, or fast food or nothing. You may feel that, on top of everything else you are supposed to get done in your busy and stressed day, you have no idea where or how to begin undoing the habits of your picky eater.

First thing to understand is that changing the habits of a picky eater will take time and will be frustrating at times. Changing any habit is a lengthy process, and as you make the changes in this book some meals will be better than others. Some days will be better than others. Trips to relatives or social occasions may feel like a set back. Vacations may throw a monkey wrench into your long hard work, and sometimes you will feel too tired or stressed to make the effort. What is helpful to understand is that there are ups and downs to anything worth doing. Factors such as time, stress and unexpected interruptions are all a part of life. If you are committed to healthy eating on a consistent basis you are making progress because this change starts with you. Then all the uncontrollable factors of life do not define your hard work and dedication to the cause.

The second thing to understand about picky eaters is their level of trust in food may be out of the ordinary. When someone eats excessive amounts of refined carbohydrates, dairy, processed oils, or refined sugars their digestive system may be out of balance. When the digestive system is out of balance the result may often be a break down in digestive health and have an affect on the way we respond to food on a mental and emotional level. A disrupted or imbalanced digestive system may have no outward signs or may be as simple as acid reflux. But, when a child under a certain age experiences digestive imbalance he or she may lack the critical thinking skills and the cognitive ability to understand what is happening in their body, as a result, they may have a limited idea that their body is not in balance. What winds up happening is food does not feel good inside them, and if the very thing that sustains our lives does not feel good, then children with digestive imbalances often crave or gravitate toward food that will fulfill them in other ways. These foods can be sweet, salty, or crunchy; or the child may insist the food does not touch on their plate, or they may have texture issues. Any one of these issues may be influenced by imbalanced digestion. The child may have developed a lack of trust for food. When there is a break down in trust, restoring trust can be difficult and will likely take patience and determination on your part. There may be a need to examine these imbalances with functional testing to help resolve the imbalances while you work on other areas.

The next piece of the puzzle is to understand exactly what a *healthy* eater looks like so that you make no mistake about what you are striving for. There is a lot of discussion in contemporary nutrition about what not to eat, whether it be gluten, dairy or meat. There are entire books written on specific subjects such as sugar, and gluten. But the reality is our busy lifestyles will take precedent for most of us unless we have a strong interest or passion in nutrition. You can learn about food in greater detail by reading my comprehensive guide book *Let's Get Real about Eating,* which is a researched and easy to read book covering multiple topics on food and food manufacturing. But, for simplification, a healthy eater does the following things:

1. Avoids artificial ingredients as much as possible; especially food dyes and high fructose corn syrup, which are the most antagonistic to a child's behavior and emotional health.
2. Makes sure any refined and processed carbohydrates eaten are as clean and wholesome as possible.
3. Eats a variety of vegetables in healthy quantities.
4. Limits the amount of refined sugar on a daily basis.

Avoiding artificial ingredients

As a parent you need to read labels. Unfortunately labels have become quite complicated to read. For the sake of the picky eater, let's simplify labels to some basics. Food coloring/food dyes are harmful to children, especially with regard to their mental and emotional well being. Read the ingredients lists to be aware of which foods contain dyes such as Red Dye, Yellow Dye and Blue Dye. These dyes are often found in kid's cereals, candy, drinks such as sports drinks, and some toothpastes. These ingredients have been found to contribute to hyperactivity in children and should be avoided as much as you can.[4] Your picky eater's behavior and emotional wellbeing gain absolutely no benefit from the consumption of food dyes. Sugars, especially refined sugars are detrimental to your child's performance as well and studies show high fructose corn syrup contributes to hyperactivity, aggression, sadness and low self-esteem.[5]

Clean and wholesome refined carbohydrates

More and more nutritional studies are presenting valuable information on the harmful effects of gluten and grains. But in keeping with the purpose of this book, it is more important that your first steps in your journey with your picky eater do not create more resistance which total gluten elimination may do. At some point you may need to eliminate gluten for other health reasons, but typically it is not a first step. Instead, rethink the quality of products containing gluten and other grains such as corn and rice. The nutritional value of gluten and other grains are significantly less when they are manufactured in combination with certain oils such as hydrogenated, regular salt over sea salt, refined sugars, and artificial ingredients like chemical preservatives. If your child consumes grains on a regular basis, it is important to stick to *whole* grains in combination with *natural* ingredients that are as clean as possible. Snack cakes, cookies, and pastries containing white flour, hydrogenated oils, and refined sugars are much more difficult for the body to break down and rank low in their nutritional value. Beware of refined carbohydrates that profess no high fructose corn syrup on the front, but still have some harmful ingredients listed on the back. For example, some cereal bars eliminate high fructose corn syrup and artificial preservatives but have hydrogenated oils and or have food dyes. Clean and wholesome carbohydrates such as bread will contain ingredients you can read and understand such as vegetable oil, honey, and yeast. It is as simple as that—if you know what to look for.

Eating enough vegetables

Eating enough vegetables does a body good. Rich in micronutrients that nourish the body, help fight illness and disease, keep us healthy and fit, vegetables are an important part of our true health. Vegetables also help our bodies deal more optimally with fruits, proteins, grains, dairy and other foods by improving the way the body breaks these foods down. Vegetables also help to neutralize the acidifying effect of proteins and grains. While complete proteins are important (some kind of complete protein should be eaten at every main meal such as eggs, fish, meat, or a legume-grain-combo), your protein is only as beneficial as the vegetables you eat throughout your day. Whether you decide to eat meat, gluten or dairy you can help keep the negative effects of any of these foods in better check if you eat enough vegetables throughout the day. Vegetables help equip the digestive system with enzymes and good fiber and micronutrients to deal with hard to digest foods such as meats, grains and cow dairy. Meats, grains and dairy are hard to digest because of the length of time it takes for the body to break these foods down from the stomach to the small intestine to the large intestine. They have become even harder to digest because of the way they are processed with antibiotics and other chemicals, or when meat is eaten with refined foods such as bread. As a result, meat, grains, and dairy are often associated with the degradation of our health. It is also important to note that fruits and vegetables are not the same thing. Eating twice as much vegetable as fruit ensures that the fruit sugars do not overstress the body by feeding sugar-eating-bacteria that lives in the digestive tract.

Limit refined sugars

Sugar is a funny subject with most parents. Often parents think they do not give their children too much sugar because soda and candy are not consumed on a daily basis. Since most of the sugar we consume is an ingredient in packaged food versus added sugar or direct sugar foods, such as candy, it is important to know your sugar. Four to five grams of sugar is equivalent to one teaspoon. If your child's breakfast cereal contains ten grams of sugar he or she starts his or her day with two full teaspoons of sugar. Eating excessive amounts of sugar is a big instigator for the picky eater to stay picky. Too much sugar can increase the taste bud's desire for more sugar perpetuating the resistance of healthier food that is naturally lower in sugar.

Most picky eaters are eating in excess of 50 grams of sugar per day. Anything over 25-30 grams of refined sugar (in packaged food, not including naturally occurring sugars like oranges and apples) will interfere in the function of healthy taste buds. If you use packaged food, you really need to strive to purchase those with around 4-5 grams (1teaspoon) of sugar per serving. If your total sugar consumption falls around 75-100 grams of sugar a day or higher, you will need to take baby steps in reducing your total sugar consumption. While implementing the strategies in later chapters, set a manageable goal of reducing your total sugar consumption by two to five grams per day until you reach a healthy amount. Each day that you successfully reduce your sugar is another day you help restore your taste buds toward enjoying healthy food.

Understand your child will still occasionally eat fast food, and participate in foods at birthday and school parties, but healthy eating on a consistent basis with good behavior provides a strong foundation making, exceptions just that. We live in a society that promotes unhealthy eating and social customs that incorporate unhealthy choices. You want your child to participate in social activities. What you do not want is a child that participates in unhealthy food so often there is no balance. You want your child to eat enough healthy foods on a consistent basis that his or her health is as strong as possible.

Keep a positive attitude as you journey forward. Some days will be better than others. Some days or even weeks can spiral you back to the beginning. But as you move through this book you will begin to change your own resolve, and the bad days will be handled differently. You will want to believe in your child's health, and this begins with your proactive involvement in his or her eating.

Tips/Summary

1. Understand the importance of eating healthy on a consistent and foundational basis.
2. Have a tough conversation with yourself and your child about the need to eat healthy.

3. Assess how much fruit and vegetables your child eats.
4. Avoid food dyes and high fructose corn syrup as much as possible.
5. Keep grains whole and wholesome with little to no artificial ingredients.
6. Believe your child should eat fruits and vegetables.
7. Understand how much refined sugar your child eats on a regular basis.
8. Limit refined sugar by decreasing appropriate amounts until desired amount is reached.
9. Allow for good days and bad days.
10. Keep a positive attitude.
11. Believe change is possible.
12. Believe in your child's nutrition as a part of your child's health.

SECRET #2

Take Ownership of Your Child's Eating

You are the greatest influence on your child.[6] Most parents understand their influence occurs up to a certain age and employ it in the areas of parenting which they feel they have the most control. In these areas, parenting comes more naturally. We all have our strengths and weaknesses as parents. This only means we are human and nothing else. When we are conscious of the areas that deserve more focus and attention, we can become better parents in those areas as well. The first step in changing the habits of a picky eater is to have a better understanding of what is out of sync with what should be happening. We have to look at the food being served. We have to look at the habits that unknowingly create picky eating behaviors. We have to look specifically at your child's behavior. Once you have a clear understanding, then we can focus on how to get your child to eat differently.

The Child's Behavior

Let's begin with some fundamental questions that will give you better understanding of what is happening and where we are going. The questions and answers below are meant to help you identify with great clarity if you have a picky eater. It is possible that your picky eater actually has more going for him or her than you realize. It is also possible that you are not quite sure if your child is a picky eater and you are just gathering information. Either way, the question and answers below will help you clarify where the problem areas lie, and present some initial strategies before we move toward larger solutions in later chapters. After you read the book in full, these questions and answers will help you reflect back to what the goals should be as you put the strategies in place.

1. What does your child eat for breakfast?

    What your child eats for breakfast is incredibly important. If your child starts his or her day with a nutritional deficit you may spend the whole day trying to get back on track to no avail. Psychology experts tell us that breakfast foods which enhance brain performance will have better brain output such as improved concentration, critical thinking and even stamina.[7] These brain foods do not have to be complicated or expensive, but can be just as simple as oatmeal with blueberries and almonds. It is very important to start your child's day off with a wholesome and healthy breakfast, his or her brain will function better and this could mean more cooperation from your child. Breakfast is also a good meal to start focusing on as you take on healthy eating.

2. Will your child eat fruit at breakfast?

    If your child will eat a piece of fruit, you can begin to improve his or her breakfast (and overall diet) by adding fresh fruit first thing in the morning. This is a great way to add a good carbohydrate, good amounts of vitamins and minerals, and does not ask the child to take too much of a risk. Most children will eat fruit before they will eat a vegetable. Breakfast is a great place to introduce eating fresh fruit and helps get your child's day off to a healthy start. This is a great first step while you take on the tougher areas in later chapters.

3. Does your child make faces or noises if presented with a fresh fruit or vegetable?

    If your child makes a face or comments negatively when faced with eating a piece of fruit or vegetable, he or she has decided long before eating the healthy food that he or she will not like it. This attitude needs to be changed in order to have a good attitude toward healthy food. A child rejecting healthy fruits and vegetables has probably spent a long time eating foods rich in sugar, salt, oil, and other ingredients that have deadened the taste buds making fresh food not nearly as pleasurable. The more healthy foods a child eats, the more their taste buds will change, and eventually healthier foods will be accepted. This kind of attitude should not be seen as a deal breaker for you, nor should it be the child's permission to avoid healthy food. So, no matter how discouraging your picky eater makes you feel, you are the parent. As you move through the strategies in this book keep putting good foods in front of him or her, especially first thing in the morning before anyone is tired from the day.

4. What does your child want to eat at snack time when given the choice?

    If your child craves the sweet and salty, then he or she has to reverse this craving and spend time cultivating healthy taste buds that have been lost along the way. Even if your child will only eat unhealthy snack food, always present a healthy choice alongside the chosen snack to help educate your child to the better choices. You can encourage a healthy snack every day swhile you work with strategies in later chapters. These chapters will present what to do at mealtime where picky eaters should not have too much freedom, but snack time is a great opportunity to present a good choice and let your child have the freedom to eat or pass on the healthy option.

5. How many times a day does your child eat half a cup of fruit and/or one-fourth a cup of vegetables?

Many parents give up trying to encourage healthy eating when they hear the requirement is four to five servings of fruit and vegetables a day. They think, "My child will never reach four or five servings, so why should I bother." Here is the key to understanding why you should bother. If your child is under the age of 10 or under 100 pounds, then a serving of fruit is ½ cup (or one piece of fruit like an apple), and a serving of vegetable is ¼ cup. Four to five servings does not mean four to five *cups* it means *servings* and not cups. Four to five servings of fruits and vegetables is a *total* of one piece of fruit and one full cup of vegetables spread out throughout the day. When you think of it like that, the end goal is not so far-fetched. As you get older the fruit serving stays the same at ½ c or one piece of fruit, but the vegetable serving increases to ½ cup.

6. Does your child take a sack lunch to school or does he or she eat the school provided lunch?

If you can pack your child's school lunch, you will have more control over what your child is eating. Having more control means having more influence, and having more influence means making greater changes. This may be challenging for some working parents. If you feel for any reason you cannot pack a lunch for your child, you will have a really hard time getting the child to manage his taste buds differently at dinner. Plus school cafeteria lunches are typically some of the most processed food your child will eat. Consider setting up a plan to help you make a lunch for your child to take to school. Making the lunch the night before can be a big help, or making the week's lunches on the weekend. If your child is old enough he or she can be a helper.

If you are having someone else prepare meals for your child, then you will need to spend time with that person to set new expectations including what ingredients or foods you expect the caretaker to use or not use. If a packed lunch is not an option for you, at least be aware of the nutritional deficit of a school prepared lunch and how much more important home meals become.

7. Does your child eat a fruit or vegetable at lunch time?

It is easy to find yourself putting into the lunch box anything and everything that comes pre-wrapped and packaged. Packaged food is often loaded with refined sugars such as high fructose corn syrup, or other harmful ingredients such as hydrogenated oils and extra sodium. Some contain food dyes or other chemical ingredients. If you are thinking about buying packaged food at a health food store, the end result may be a higher grocery bill and not necessarily better nourishment only less offensive ingredients. An organic cookie may have less harmful ingredients and may be a better choice of cookie, but it does not replace the wholesome fruit or vegetable serving. You do not have to break the bank or slave in the kitchen to get something wholesome in your child's lunchbox. Take a few seconds and put some baby carrots in a small plastic baggie, or small container. Cut up an apple and put it in a baggie. You can add a small damp paper towel to help keep the fruit from browning. Make sure your child is accustomed to having a fruit and or vegetable in the lunch box. Of course, the fruit or vegetable may come back home while you are putting later strategies in place. This is common. Helpful suggestions may be to serve the fruit or vegetable with a dip, such as apples and peanut butter, strawberries and yogurt, cucumber and salad dressing, broccoli and maple syrup to help the fruit or vegetable be eaten instead of ignored. Make sure if you are using dips or dressings you look at the grams of sugar.

8. Does your child *leave* the dinner table without eating what is prepared and help him or herself to a snack an hour or so later?

Picky eaters manifest is many ways. Rejecting prepared meals and sneaking snack food is another way a child escapes the healthy food and satisfies his or her desires. As you begin this journey to help improve the eating habits of your picky eater, it is important to realize the picky eater is more about behavior than anything else. Change is sometimes difficult, but with persistence you can help create change. Your picky eater is not a picky eater by birth. Most picky eaters are learned picky eaters. And the change begins now.

Some Things to Think About

Now that we know some of the characteristics of a picky eater, let's consider how our own behavior might be contributing to our picky eater's resistance to healthy foods. Below are a few questions that will help you identify whether or not you might have to look at your own behavior. If you answer yes to one or more of these questions you will be asked in later chapters to understand your role in the life of your picky eater.

But remember, even if some of your own behavior is unknowingly contributing to your picky eater by taking action you demonstrate your commitment to your child is far greater.

1. Do you reach for junk food or alcohol after work, before dinner and in front of your child?

   Be careful what you are modeling in front of your child. If you reach for a certain kind of food or alcohol to deal with certain mental or emotional stresses you are sending a harmful subliminal message to your child. You may be sending a message that managing stress is done through food and drink, which defeats the purpose of food as nutrition. Modeling good eating behavior is crucial and is discussed in greater detail in a later chapter.

2. Do you watch television while eating or answer your phone at mealtime in front of your child?

   In order to be successful eliminating picky eater behaviors, you will have to make mealtime a priority. You will need to make his or her behavior at the table your priority. If you are distracted with phone calls or the television, you send a message to your picky eater that they are not important enough. Distracted behavior on the part of the parent can also instigate negative attention-seeking behaviors from the child.

3. Do you sneak junk food when you think no one is looking?

You would be surprised what your child knows and does not know about you. They may not know what is in your bank account, but you can be sure they have a pretty good idea of what you are eating. You cannot move through this book trying to take away candy from their diets while hiding it in the back of the pantry for your own indulgence at a later time. Forgive yourself if this is your pattern, but also think about the need for collective change.

4. Do you reward or punish your child with food?

Food as a reward can contribute to unhealthy eating habits and poor boundaries. Consider whether or not you offer sugar enhanced foods as a reward for eating other foods, or whether you withhold sugar treats as a consequence. Sugar foods as a reward or to motivate your child toward healthy eating will only perpetuate a subconscious distaste for healthy foods. A child could easily come to believe, "Sugar as reward equals good, vegetable as the means to the good must equal bad." See how that undermines your ultimate effort?

Here is the bottom line: We are what we eat. We put food into our bodies that either contains nutrients or does not contain nutrients. Either there is quality fuel to run the body and the brain, or there is not. Food is not just about our pleasure centers, or our stressful schedules, instead food is about who we are and how we perform. Food is also related to the health and fitness of our body, which is connected to how we view our bodies which is connected to our self esteem. If we have a poor view of our bodies then we may have a poor sense of self.[8]

Many of you are spending a small fortune in extra-curricular activities for your children to help them excel, yet we spend less and less on the food that fuels their bodies and converts directly into the quality of their performance. And even less attention is given to eating healthy as a part of a healthy view of one's self. It is time to consider food as part of the formula that helps put your child at the top of his or her game—mentally, emotionally and physically.

SECRET #3

Have a Nutritional Value System

Most parents enforce homework. Homework is a necessary part of school. Most of you do not let your child escape doing homework. It is not a choice they get to make. If they have homework, they have to do it. Going to school and doing homework is important to you because you have a strong commitment, as part of your value system, to your child's education. You care about what kind of child you are raising, and what kind of adult you hope he or she will become. If you attend church, you may view religion similarly to education. Or maybe you have a stronger commitment to your child's morality and spiritual development over education. Either way you have placed value on certain things in your child's life. What you may have failed to see, thus far, is the connection between your child's personal developments, both academically and spiritually, with what they eat. There is a strong connection between what your child eats and how they perform.

This human body that we occupy is an amazing machine. This body makes new cells every day as old cells die, or to replace damaged cells. Even the cells in our brain. This happens millions of times a day.

Some of this process, called the cell cycle, is influenced by the raw materials we give our body. This raw material is otherwise known as food. This means that the quality of food we eat has a direct bearing on what kind of person we are. As a result, we really are what we eat. If we are what we eat, then the education of our children is somewhat dependent on the quality of food they consume. If we really are what we eat, regulating the chemical balances and imbalances that form our emotional wellbeing with food, then our morality and ability to be the best we can be is dependent not just on a personal relationship with God but also on our ability to be the best version of ourselves. What we eat then becomes a big part of our spirituality as well.

If we can understand the need for quality whole foods as an integral part of becoming the best version of ourselves then healthy eating is right up there with our child's education and spiritual development. Once we understand this link and believe it to be true, we can make a commitment to healthy eating as a necessary value we teach in the home. Once we are committed to eating well, then we can more readily stay committed when our child wants macaroni and cheese over broccoli. We can then have a strong fundamental connection with eating an apple over eating a cookie every day.

If you are married, it is very important to have a united front. Just as you have conversations about religion, education, politics, places to live, and other topics that directly impact your lives and the lives of your children, it is very important to consider nutrition part of your health and, in doing so, make it a consideration just as important as your religion, your politics, or your education. It does not mean you have to agree on everything, but you should agree on a platform that helps you collectively raise your children. If you do this, then no one parent has to be the food police. A united front in the face of a picky eater prevents the picky eater from wedging himself or herself between two parents that shifts the focus away from the child's nutrition and toward the family's dynamics. A united front also prevents indulging in bad food when the "nutritional" parent is absent. Instead, the focus can be on resolving the picky eater behavior.

It is crucial to come to a working agreement and commit to key nutritional decisions as a couple when the children are *not* present. You may decide that your family will only drink sodas on the weekend, or when on vacation. Then, when the child is begging for soda either parent can give the guideline, "we only drink soda on the weekend" as opposed to "mommy said no" or "sure, your mom is not here." This also helps what goes in the grocery cart no matter who goes to the grocery store. Here are some sample questions to help determine your nutritional value system going forward.

1. How often do we eat fast food and when?
2. How often do we drink soda and when?
3. How much candy do we eat and how often?
4. When do we eat dessert?
5. When do we eat junk food?
6. When is it most important to eat healthy food?
7. What are the guidelines about eating what is served on our plate?
8. What is the rule when going to someone else's house?
9. What should our children know about birthday parties and sleepovers relative to eating?

The answers to these questions become your guidelines and make a strong statement that our food choices are important because they have a big impact on our health and wellbeing as opposed to the battle for power between two parents. These guidelines help give you and your spouse a common language that informs decisions from the grocery store, to picking up dinner, to a night out. Eventually, you want your child to make good choices when you are not around. This is especially true if the picky eater is trying to assert control over the parent. Creating a value system with guidelines means there can be no control over a parent. There is only control over the choices we make surrounding food.

Tips/Summary

1. Understand the importance of what your existing family values are such as education and religion.

SECRET #4

Motivate Your Child

W e expect children to follow certain rules. They have to go to school, do their homework, and go to church, just to name a few. Many parents also ask their children to do certain tasks around the house. Many parents will pay their children an allowance or keep a responsibility chart to keep their child motivated to do some of these tasks. If you have some kind of system in place for your child's household responsibilities, then you have a basic understanding of what is necessary to motivate your child. Without some expectation and motivation most children would spend the day in front of the television or video games and not lift a finger to help around the house.

If children are designed to avoid responsibility unless strongly motivated to do so, why do we expect healthy eating to be any less enticing? Given that most parents have very clear cut expectations for their children regarding things such as going to school, going to church, even cleaning up their room, it is time to consider clear cut expectations on healthy eating too. Without clear expectations there may be too much freedom to choose what they will and will not eat. In doing so, most parents do not understand that they are contributing to their child being a "picky eater." Given the choice between ice cream and broccoli, what would you chose? Picky eaters have become picky eaters for many reasons, and unfortunately one of those reasons is they were allowed to become a picky eater. And they will not get anywhere else unless we as parents change our view of the *expectation and motivation* of eating healthy.

We are all driven by either extrinsic or intrinsic motivation. Extrinsic motivation comes from a source outside of us like points scored while playing a sport, getting good grades in school, earning money to buy things or afford a particular kind of vacation. Intrinsic motivation comes from within us. When we discover just doing something is reward enough, we are experiencing intrinsic motivation. One example would be playing a game without keeping score.

As parents we realize that there are certain behaviors that require either a reward or a consequence. If your child does not do his or her homework and receives a poor grade, there may be a significant consequence at home for his or her failure to follow through on set expectations. As we watch our children change and evolve each year, we begin to adapt our parenting based on the child's personality. For example, you may have a child that will brush his or her teeth without being told or requiring a reward or consequence while a different child may not. In some cases, maturity will change the child's desire to brush his teeth without being told, but in the meantime you have a child that will not brush his or her teeth. If you have to reinforce your parenting with a reward or consequence, you are using extrinsic motivation to encourage your child to meet the expectation.

Somehow, when it comes to eating healthy, we assume the child should automatically want to eat vegetables. If it is good for us, we should just want to eat it. Or the child may have had a healthy appetite as a baby, and we cannot understand the change in his or her behavior. When we assume the child should just want to eat healthy, we are expecting intrinsic motivation to happen in the area of healthy eating. Most adults eat healthy because they believe there is a correlation between healthy eating and their health or their weight, or they are avoiding certain symptoms by avoiding certain foods. By doing this, adults are using extrinsic motivation to encourage their own healthy eating. Very few adults are eating healthy foods consistently out of pure pleasure (intrinsically). Why are we expecting our children to do differently?

It is important to align the expectations you set for your child with the proper motivation—extrinsic. The best way to approach healthy eating with extrinsic motivation is to create incentive with appropriate reward non-food rewards. Since a negative attitude already exists within a picky eater, motivation and reinforcement based on a negative consequence does not help encourage a positive attitude toward healthy food. Working towards something is far better than running away from something. This even holds true for adults. It is better to eat healthy as a preventative measure, than to eat healthy later on to relieve pain or lose weight. So now is the time to lay down a healthy foundation for your child that he or she can carry with them throughout their adult lives. This foundation will even help them have a positive self esteem. Each phase of maturity will require different kinds of motivation.

Toddler Years (Age 2-4)

Toddlers often behave positively to visual stimulation and lots of bright color. Try these suggestions for motivating your toddler to eat healthy foods.

Party Time

Use a collection of simple party hats, and other inexpensive party type favors to motivate your toddler at the table. Some good party hats are crowns and tiaras, which can include the dialogue of being a king or a princess when you eat healthy and take care of your body. Hats can stay in a basket at the table and come on and off for mealtime only. If they are worn outside of mealtime they will lose their significance to the meal itself. Another key to this strategy working is to have everyone in the family participate no matter their age. Anyone at the table who eats their vegetables gets to wear the party hat. Here is why it is important for everyone to participate. If the picky eater continues to resist the healthy food, which is usually vegetables, he will see other family members, including mom and dad being recognized and honored with the party hats. And he or she may give in after a time since he or she will not want to feel left out.

Other decorative items such as fancy rings or necklaces can also be a token of honor for eating healthy foods. Any shiny or colorful object that you can connect to be honored can be used. Again, needs to stay in a basket or box at the table and used only to motivate and encourage healthy eating. Again, everyone should participate to add pressure to the picky eater so that he or she will want to be included. You can even go so far has to have party noisemakers that can be made to make the celebratory noise every time the child eats his complete serving of the resistant food.

Young Years (Age 5-9)

During these years, children are learning about setting and achieving goals. You can help them learn to set and achieve healthy eating habits through the following reward-based ideas.

Healthy Eating Sticker Chart

Create a sticker chart like the one pictured at the back of this book, or if you prefer you can print one for free at www.laurakopec.com or find the chart on my Facebook page. If you make your own, be sure to include a bonus spot for trying a new food. You can also encourage more ownership by having your child actually make the sticker chart, or color and add designs to a formatted one that has a grid. A sticker chart showing one week at a time works more effectively to establish both daily and end-of-the-week goals. Then decide on corresponding rewards: a daily reward for daily accomplishments and a weekly reward for a full week of progress.

Make sure you set your child up for success by setting the bar on the first day within his or her reach. For example, if your child has an easy time with fruits and protein, but struggles with vegetables you can say, "You have to get two stickers every day to get your daily reward." This way the child is sure to get at least two stickers from eating protein and fruit. Then expect more the next day or subsequent days once the child has a taste of achieving the daily reward. By keeping the expectation manageable on the first couple of days, the child gets a quick taste of success and knows what he or she has to do next. It is important to establish a time frame for your child to get a sticker in the resistant-food box. For example, if day one and two were easy stickers, now day three or four has to have a sticker on the resistant food to get the daily reward. The reward should *never* be food, especially dessert or junk food, and does not have to be a material object. Provide some incentive that is time based such as an extra story at story time, or fifteen minutes of computer time. If the child refuses to eat the resistant food, then he or she does not get his sticker and does not get the daily reward.

Then set the expectation for the week such as at least three stickers on four of the seven days to earn the end-of-week-reward. This establishes a long-term goal which is a reward he or she can achieve by the end of the week. The end-of-the-week reward should be a bit more significant than the daily reward such as trip to the park or a trip to the library or a movie. Use your own knowledge of your child to create a reward he or she will be inclined to strive for. Avoid rewards that do not matter to the child. Some children will work for story time, while others will not care about stories. Some children will do anything for a video game, while others will not care about video games. The sticker chart is only as effective as the reward is valuable to the child.

Create a Healthy Body Collage

Similar to the Healthy Sticker Chart, the Healthy Body Collage is a learning tool as well and may be something you want to use more than a sticker chart for an older child. You can create an outline of the human body with a representation of a brain, muscles, organs and skeleton. Then have some pictures of healthy foods and match up the area of the body that they go to. For example, a picture of walnuts, almonds, blueberries, salmon, and cauliflower can go over the brain. Pictures of almonds, yogurt, and soybeans can go over bones. Green beans, spinach, salmon, and oatmeal can go over the heart, carrots over the eyes and peaches over the skin. Super foods that help the entire body such as kale, spinach, and broccoli can be placed anywhere.

You can personalize the Healthy Body Collage by using a photo of your child on a poster board with healthy food items to stick on his or her body. If personalized, take the opportunity to also have your child write descriptive adjectives that describe your child's positive traits. This gives your child a strong personal connection to the collage and over time imprint the entire visual into his or her brain where it will have a strong connection.

For advanced learners, you can make the Healthy Body Collage a research project with your child where you take a list of healthy foods and they have to find out what part of the body those foods help. Or you can keep it less intense and just ask them to come up with a list of healthy foods that help make the body healthy—placing those pictures anywhere on the body. You can even go further and put a picture of a trash can in the corner, and put some pictures of food that do harm to the body such as drinks containing food dyes, cakes containing hydrogenated oils, and packaged foods containing high fructose corn syrup inside the trash can where they belong.

A Note about Rewards

If the child earns the reward, do not take the reward away when the child does something wrong in another area. Consequences for one behavior should never involve taking away rewards given previously for good behavior. If a child earned something, then he or she earned it. If you give and then you take away what was given, you completely undermine the child's desire and motivation. Then they will always think, "why bother if it can be just as easily taken away."

Pre-Teen and Early Teen Years (10-14)

The preteen and early teen years are crucial because by the time a child is fifteen years old, he or she will believe they are an adult and capable of making their own decisions even though he or she is not really an adult. Picky eating habits that have been present for years and years are very difficult to break if the teenager is unwilling. Certainly the earlier you can work with a child the better, but the last window of opportunity is during these pre-teen years. A few strategies can help motivate this age group.

Ticket Jar

By age ten or eleven, your child can handle combining rewards for multiple kinds of good behavior. A ticket jar works best when used as a reward for many responsibilities and can be used to teach some basic money management skills indirectly, so it has dual purpose. Purchase some simple raffle tickets at your local department or office supply store. Make a list of all responsibilities or behaviors that will be rewarded with tickets. Next, determine how many tickets each responsibility or behavior will earn. Tickets are given every time behavior is worthy of being recognized. This allows for you to have some say about the quality of work/attitude while earning tickets.

Of course, a corresponding plan to redeem tickets needs to be in place. Create on a sheet of paper what tickets are worth. For example, five tickets may equal thirty minutes of video games, ten tickets for a trip to the mall, fifteen tickets equals a trip to the movies. You should even create a larger reward for twenty-five tickets. You get to decide. Then at the end of the week, you can sit down and redeem tickets. The great thing is your child gets to decide if he or she wants to redeem tickets, how many he or she wants to redeem or if tickets should be saved for the bigger reward. By "saving" or "spending" tickets, he or she gets to learn indirectly about money too.

Junior Chef

As your child matures, you can assign a meal to your preteen or teenager to plan, prepare and serve all on his or her own. Make sure the meal is age appropriate. The ten-year-old may need to be in charge of a weekend lunch where the meal can be cold foods in order to avoid using the oven or stove. As the advance in years, you can increase the level of difficulty. By the age of fourteen, most young adults can handle some basic meals such as French toast, grilled cheese sandwiches with tomato soup, hamburger patties with baked French fries and salad, or mini-homemade pizzas with salad. You will have to teach them and involve them in the kitchen as an assistant before you give them the reins; but at some point, they should earn the right and the responsibility of a meal. Make sure you educate him or her on what your expectations are for the meal. The meal should contain a source of protein, and at least one vegetable. With a greater sense of independence based on clear expectations, your child may be inspired and motivated, at the very least, to eat what they prepared.

No matter what age or where your child is starting in his or understanding of eating healthy, you can have a positive motivation program in place to help inspire a desire for healthy eating. Use wise parenting decisions to set appropriate expectations within the motivation program and give appropriate rewards. Make changes as you see fit to help continually inspire and motivate your child. Expect the extrinsic motivation to be in place for several months to ensure ownership of good eating habits.

Tips/Summary

1. Avoid unrealistic expectations of your child.
2. Realize your child will not eat healthy for the sake of eating healthy.
3. Realize healthy eating is not intrinsic and will take some extrinsic motivation.
4. Utilize age-appropriate strategies for motivating your child to eat healthy foods.
5. Set short-term and long-term goals.
6. Avoid taking away an earned reward as a consequence.
7. Make sure the reward is truly important to your child or it will fail as a motivator.
8. Avoid food rewards.

9. Toddler strategies include Party Time with hats and favors.
10. Younger-year strategies include Healthy Sticker Chart and Body Collage.
11. Preteen and teen strategies include Ticket Jar and Junior Chef.

SECRET # 5

Establish Family Mealtime

We are by far a busier generation of families than previous generations. When I was growing up in the 70's and early 80's after school activities or sports happened directly after school and everyone was home for dinner. It was unheard of to have a practice that ran to 7:00 or 8:00 pm at night. It was unheard of that dinner would be had at the drive through window on the way to this practice or that game. It was unheard of that mom or dad would stop to pick up dinner on the way home for work. I lived in a different time and that family lifestyle is at least two generations past. Now we are fast paced, overextended and stressed. Our lifestyle now is very different than the lifestyle of my childhood. In order to have healthy eating habits, we have to look at our current lifestyle and what can be done within its parameters with all its stresses and complications. And even though our current parenting style and type of child rearing differs so completely from previous generations studies show there were some benefits to previous parenting styles.

The family dinner has long been professed to do so much more than just serve a home cooked meal. It is a time for coming together, for having conversation, for knowing what has gone on in your child's day. The family dinner encourages healthy self-esteem and a strong sense of security in the family unit. Without traditional routines such as family dinner, it is possible our children are coming up short not only on quality family time but also in their very development. Studies at Cornell University show that children that have family dinner time have a greater chance of eating healthier foods and will be more likely to avoid eating disorders and obesity.[9] It goes even beyond eating though. According to research at Purdue University, children who participate in family mealtime are more likely to be successful academically and have a better vocabulary.[10] Children who participate in family mealtime are less likely to smoke and engage in recreational drugs.[11] Not only is family mealtime good for your children, but studies show family mealtime can help relieve stress in adults, especially in women.[12] It is clear that family mealtime is important for everyone, and at the very least has to be adapted to fit our busy lifestyles.

You can take your first step toward family mealtime that fits your current lifestyle. First, find at least one night a week that you can gather at the dinner table for a family meal. At that dinner, it needs to be very clear that family mealtime means the focus is on the family. This means no interruptions once the meal has started. No one should be allowed to take even a phone call once dinner has started. This meal should be as wholesome as possible, even if it is prepared somewhere else. That means there should be no bags or wrappers at the table. Even if the meal was prepared somewhere else, leave all the wrappers in the kitchen and put the food on plates and bring the meal to the table.

Then use family mealtime to have positive conversation. In addition to developing your child's conversation skills, you can influence their eating habits. When positive conversation and feel good emotions are present while eating, there is the strong likelihood of developing a strong association of healthy food with good feelings and good times. For example, if someone just mentions certain Thanksgiving food such as roasted turkey, stuffing, cranberry sauce and pumpkin pie most people conjure up a good feeling. Positive conversations at mealtime include asking questions about your child's day, knowing the other children they spend their social time with and helping guide your child toward having gratitude about their day.

Next, make mealtime a no-tech zone. Even if mealtime is on the go, it should never be combined with phones, video games, or television. Once in a while, it is fine to have a meal in front of the television or movie, but the combination of eating with phones, videos or television is counterproductive to healthy eating habits and is also really distressing to the digestive system. Many people change the pace of their eating mindlessly chewing at a pace similar to the activity or conversation on the screen and fail to eat consciously. That is why many people overeat when eating in front of the television. Even in adults, eating in front of the television has been shown to contribute to weight gain.

Lastly, establish the importance of eating with thoughtfulness and consciousness. Family mealtime is a time to nourish your body with good things, pay attention to eating, and have conversations with those around you. It is a great time to have positive and encouraging conversations about healthy eating as well. Purdue University created a great acronym for family mealtime: Family Meals spell SUCCESS.[13]

S – Smarter children
U – Unlikely to smoke
C – Courteous and conversational
C – Connected to family
E – Eating better
S – Sharing food and conversation
S – Strengthen families

Eating healthy is not just what we put in our mouth, but how we treat the mealtime itself.

Tips/Summary

1. Understand the importance of family mealtime.

2. Establish family mealtime by having a family dinner. Even if this can only happen once a week. Be consistent and ritualistic about that time.
3. Practice once a week, until you feel comfortable adding another family mealtime.
4. Consider good presentation of the food as part of the respect for the meal and the time together as a family.
5. Have positive conversation about your child's day.
6. Make family mealtime a no-tech zone. No phones, videos, television or computers during family mealtime.
7. Eat with a positive attitude and togetherness remembering that family mealtime equals SUCCESS.

SECRET #6

Model Good Behavior

One of the most important strategies for getting your child to have a more well-rounded and healthy diet is for you, the parent, to eat a well-rounded and healthy diet. Plain and simple, parents need to model good eating. Children are incredibly smart and very perceptive. If you are asking them to do something that you are not doing, then there is a very good chance they will refuse to do it. There is an inherent ability for children to spot hypocrisy and rebel against it. Parents that model good eating habits are far more likely to help a picky eater become a better eater than parents that do not.

Many adults feel that, by the time they are adults, they should be able to eat whatever they want. However, when you become a parent, it becomes even more critical that you model appropriately for your children in all areas. Research on parenting and discipline in recent years places greater importance on parental influence than ever before.[14] The saying, "do as I say, not as I do" is becoming archaic as we understand that no matter what we say, our children are more likely to model our behavior than follow our instructions. This carries over to food as well. Studies show children's taste in food is influenced by watching the food choices of other influencing persons such as parents, teachers and even peers.[15] We cannot control the choices of teachers and peers, but we can control our own choices and have the greater influence on our children.

It is also important to have healthy conversations with your child about role models, all kinds of role models.[16] You can encourage children to have positive role models and discuss the characteristics of what makes a positive role model. You can also discuss how sometimes a role model can make a mistake. According to the American Academy of Child and Adolescent Psychiatry, it is important to realize our children will have role models and to talk to our children about their role models through positive conversation.[17] Being able to discuss the mistakes of a role model can also help a parent, who previously made poor eating choices, turn over a new leaf and focus on the positive changes in eating that are happening for everyone.

If you are constantly asking your child to eat healthy foods because everyone in the family is expected to eat healthy foods, cooperation is more likely to happen. Consistency is important, but this does not mean you have to be a perfect eater, exceptions teach children appropriateness to the norm. But, it is crucial that you eat healthy, not only for your success with your picky eater but also for your own good health. Healthy eating is then something that everyone does because it is good for them, and no one is singled out. When healthy eating is modeled by everyone, your positive parenting messages are reinforced through example.

Tips/Summary

1. Consider your influence on your child.
2. Understand your child will place a premium on role models.
3. Be a positive role model for your child in eating.
4. Have a positive conversation about role models and mistakes.
5. Set an example for your child by modeling healthy eating.
6. Encourage healthy eating for the whole family.

SECRET #7

Celebrate Good Food

We have a tendency in our society to connect special times with unhealthy food options. For example, birthday parties typically serve pizza, cake and ice cream. Soccer matches finish at fast food places. The convenience, the prices and the obvious enjoyment are hard to resist. There is a very good chance these kinds of associations will continue in our current society. The problem is when the *only* connection we make between good times and food is unhealthy eating. We need to be conscious of the fact that healthy eating needs to have some chance of being associated with good times.

There are opportunities to incorporate good times with healthy eating. If those opportunities are not readily available, you can create them. One type of event you can create is to have a healthy picnic. You can specifically plan an outing that is focused on good times and healthy food. Pack some fresh fruit, whole grain crackers, cheese, along with some time at the playground or lake to make the event fun.

Another suggestion is for a family Sunday outing to a healthier restaurant. Making a specific point to go to a healthy restaurant as a family sends a good message about quality time and family time. Combining this with going to church as a family further reinforces the positive message of church, family and health. If money is a concern, consider going for breakfast or lunch, since many restaurants have less expensive breakfasts and lunches.

Another suggestion is to have a homemade pizza party. Have each person make a personal pizza picking the toppings they want. You can have the toppings set up buffet style where everyone gets to put their own toppings onto the pizza sauce and cheese. You can add to the experience by playing fun music or making a game of who uses the most colorful toppings (including vegetables).

Another suggestion is intentionally planning a healthy potluck with another family that allows friends to share their healthy recipes with each other. Barbeque or pool parties are another way of creating a healthy and social potluck.

Another suggestion is to have a Family Member's Pick Night where everyone in the family take turns picking a menu with preset healthy considerations for a particular night of the week. For example, on the first Saturday of the month, it is Dad's turn to pick a dinner that contains at least one cooked vegetable and a salad of some kind. The next Saturday, it is your child's turn and so on.

Studies show that eating habits are strongly associated with traditions and social customs.[18] If we were raised with healthy customs, it is our responsibility to carry some of those customs and traditions on to the next generation. If we were not raised with healthy customs, then it is our opportunity and responsibility to create rituals and customs to which our children can feel a connection to healthy eating.

Tips/Summary

1. Recognize how often good times happen in conjunction with unhealthy eating.
2. Make a decision to incorporate some healthy eating with good times.
3. Have a healthy family picnic.

4. Combine church with a healthy restaurant and family meal before or after.
5. Throw a homemade pizza party.
6. Have a healthy potluck with family and/or friends.
7. Have Family Member's Pick Night, where a different member gets to pick dinner.
8. Celebrate events with good food.

SECRET #8

Make One Meal

We all want to be good parents. Just the fact that you are reading this book indicates you are a devoted parent that is interested in making improvements in your family. Somehow many of us believe that catering to our children's likes and dislikes is healthy for their development. We need to remember we are raising young children into adults. What does an adult look like whose life is based on his or her likes and dislikes? Possibly a very unhappy adult, since healthy and responsible adulthood does not revolve around our likes and dislikes. While adult eating presents us with the possibility of always eating what we like and always avoiding what we dislike, the truth is sometimes what is good for us is not always what we like.

It is amazing how many parents of picky eaters are making two or more meals. One meal is made for the non-picky family members and then one meal for each picky eater. Often the parent who is making a special meal for their picky eater does so under the notion that the child "won't eat anything else." The parent believes that the child would starve if they did not prepare a diet of their favorite foods. Picky eaters may become defensive and stubborn, but you have to be willing to take that first step for his or her success. Have a healthy mindset for yourself first by preparing one meal. Believe it is acceptable to make one healthy meal and expect your child to eat what you cook. Then realize it takes on average ten to fifteen times of eating new food before your picky eater will incorporate the food into his or her daily regime. If you never present the food, he or she is never given the pathway to success.

It is perfectly acceptable to have boundaries as the caretaker and make *one* meal. There are subliminal messages to everything we say and do. Remember our children are more likely to model our behavior as adults than do the opposite. When you make one meal, you establish that you are a hard working parent that sees each family member as part of a team where everyone eats the same meal. When you make a specific meal for your picky eater, this says you are not just a hard working parent, but a short order cook who serves the individual requests of the family. A special meal for the picky eater says family members are not team players as a family should be. The special meal for the picky eater places focus on the individual over what is healthy and wholesome for the entire family.

Making more than one meal is an easy trap to fall into. It may seem to make life easier if you have a strong-willed child, but you are actually creating more of a problem with each special meal. Restaurants are the time we get to choose from a selection, home cooked meals are not the time we should get to choose. Even if your child has special dietary needs, you should make one meal. The child with special dietary needs should feel like the home cooked meal includes his or health specifications, but does not set him or her up to be an outcast at family mealtime. The child with special needs already feels excluded in his or her peer group and does not need to feel this at home. It is appropriate to have two different kinds of bread if one child has to be gluten free, and the gluten free bread is too expensive for the whole family. Making the same meal with two kinds of bread is fine, but having pizza and making the gluten-free child have tacos is not okay.

The overall message of one meal says we are all to be treated equally as much as possible during family mealtime. Serving one meal says the focus is on our family's nutrition and well-being. Preparing and serving one meal sends a message that the person cooking is sharing their gifts and talents, and helps enforce the idea of unity in the kitchen. Individual tastes can still accompany a one-meal dinner. Condiments, salt and pepper, salad dressing, etc. can be used to the taste and preference of individuals at the table. This allows individuals to make choices on how they want to customize their *one* meal, but does not cater to the individual with a completely different meal.

If the picky eater refuses to eat the meal you serve, it is appropriate to tell the child that when he or she is hungry enough they can join in the meal being served. It is important to establish you are *not* keeping food from the child instead you are taking the position that you are not a short order cook. You can wrap the plate, keep it warm—whatever you need to do to show love and care, except giving the child an out which only reinforces an unhealthy exception for the picky eater. If the picky eater refuses what is on the table with the knowledge that he or she can get a bowl of cereal an hour or so later, or warm up something in the microwave, or have cookies or crackers than all you have done is give them permission to refuse your cooking the next time. Only by staying strong, having appropriate boundaries at mealtime, and holding the position of one healthy meal for all can you make a difference in the picky eater who refuses to eat.

Tips/Summary

1. Avoid making more than one meal for the same mealtime.
2. Have complimentary condiments available with each meal to allow individuals to customize their own meal.
3. If a meal is refused, keep the meal ready for when the picky eater is hungry.
4. Avoid allowing the picky eater to refuse a meal then eat something else later.
5. Stand by your decision of one meal and eating what is made.
6. Understand one meal reinforces family community and unity.

SECRET #9

Empower Your Child

The more involved and connected someone feels to someone or something, the more important that person or thing is to the individual. Therefore, the more involved your child is with other aspects of food such as grocery shopping, understanding food, and making good food choices, the more important eating healthy will become to your child. When empowered with the ability to be involved, the more entrusted he or she will feel.

If your child is between the age of four and ten, you can create a collage of healthy foods that you want your child to eat called a Choosing Chart. A wide variety of healthy fruits and vegetables, healthy proteins and healthy snacks should make up the collage. You can download images from the computer, or you can use old magazines. Use construction paper and have your child be creative choosing healthy foods, especially the ones he or she does like, or the ones he or she is willing to try. Then when you make your weekly grocery list, you can ask your child to choose from the Choosing Chart what items should be added to the grocery cart. You can also use the chart for reinforcement by letting your child put a sticker on the item every time he or she eats that particular food. Remember the Choosing Chart should only have healthy options.

If your child is older than ten years, you may use or create a different kind of Choosing Chart. Older kids when given the complete project will be creative and imaginative, so ask your child to create an entire project demonstrating healthy foods he or she likes. If your child is reluctant to create something from scratch, you can ask your child to use a food pyramid chart which is a better start than not having any guidelines.

Next, take your child grocery shopping. Most parents will chose to grocery shop alone without the pressure and stress of children alongside. But take a moment to rethink the grocery store. Not only is it a place to purchase the essentials, but it is also a classroom. Time can still be precious, so making a list in advance of getting to the store allows you more time to encourage participation from your child. Play a grocery store game and have them do the following:

1. Find a snack without food dyes. (Teach readers to look for words like Red Dye #40; and for non-readers, point out the visual difference between snacks with food dyes and snacks without.)
2. Find a snack without high fructose corn syrup (for readers).
3. Find a snack that is wholesome and healthy (for readers and non-readers).

If your child was the "grocery shopper" and picked out some of the food to go into the cart, they will take pride in their purchases. You also have a future card to play – they made the choice at the store – if they refuse to eat their choice.

You can also teach your child how to choose produce. Teach your child how to look for apples with no bruises or dents or cuts in the skin. Talk to him or her about how different apples can have different flavors and maybe you can try a different apple for a new experience. He or she might find a new favorite with the opportunity to experiment with healthy food. If your child is more creative and artistic, you can encourage the creative side by asking him or her to put as many colors of the rainbow in the shopping cart. If your child is more structured and needs things ordered and precise, you can ask him or her to do more of the counting and bagging. Ask for a specific amount of apples to be put in a produce bag. Remember use numbers and weights more than colors to involve your structured and ordered child in the grocery store. Use more colors and creativity to involve your creative and free-spirited child.

Overall, the goal is to involve your child with the planning part of eating. Learning about food, finding a new recipe, making a list, helping make good choices in the grocery store is all part of the empowerment. If your child is involved in the planning stage, he or she will feel like there is ownership of the food even before sitting down to eat.

Tips/Summary

1. Consider involving your child in grocery shopping and understanding good food choices.
2. Create a Choosing Chart for empowering your child to choose healthy foods.
3. Ask your child to contribute to the grocery list.
4. Take your child grocery shopping on occasion.
5. Ask the creative child to choose colorful foods.
6. Ask the structured child to help count and bag produce of other healthy foods.
7. Encourage even more involvement in the planning stage.

SECRET #10

Create a Helper Not a Rebel

Another great way to increase your child's involvement, which will improve their ownership, is to involve your child in the preparation and ritual of mealtime. Being connected to the preparation is just like the anticipation of a party. There is great excitement and emotional investment in the anticipation of an event. The younger the child the more interested he or she might be in helping. Older children's interest may depend on the presentation of the idea. Use a positive tone when inviting your child to help, this will send a positive subconscious message that helping is a privilege and not a chore.

Choose appropriate tasks based on the age of the child. A three- or four-year-old can help stir a mixing bowl filled with ingredients. A five- and six-year-old can help pour measured out ingredients into the bowl and stir items. A seven- and eight-year-old can help get ingredients out of the refrigerator or pantry, can help measure certain ingredients you are comfortable having them measure, and can pour and mix. Depending on your child's maturity a ten- to twelve-year-old can peel vegetables, stir ingredients on the stove top and do tasks such as flip pancakes and know when liquid is boiling. You can give some basics to your preteen from start to finish such as making scrambled eggs. A teenager can begin to do complete tasks, such as making a salad, a side dish or even a dessert. And once your child is fifteen or sixteen he or she should have the job of a full meal preparation if they have been properly instructed.

At some point after graduating from high school your children will find themselves having the responsibility of grocery shopping and meal preparation. Will they be equipped for this enormous task or will they be forced to either learn the hard way or avoid learning by eating mostly restaurant food? The average weight gain during four years of college is approximately 40 lbs affecting not just a small number of students, but 70% of all college students.[19] Gone is the previous "Freshman 15" weight gain which used to affect only a small portion of college students. This weight gain happens for many reasons, but one reason is that grocery shopping and meal preparation are not skills we are teaching our children before they leave home. If you have a teenager at home, you might want to sit down and think about some of the basic skills they should know by the time they leave for college. When it comes to meals, make a basic list of what you want your teenager to know. Examples are

1. Roasting a chicken,
2. Making spaghetti,
3. Steaming broccoli,
4. Making banana bread,
5. Baking a potato,
6. Making a basic tossed salad, and
7. Making turkey burgers.

If you can teach your teenager seven to twelve different basic meals they can make without recipes, they will be much more equipped to continue eating healthy after leaving home. If you can teach them the importance of fruits and vegetables at every meal they are more likely to think before they eat.

Another important helper skill is setting the table. Children can start helping to set the table as early as four years old. Begin with appropriate items such as spoons and napkins, and avoid glassware and knives until they are mature and demonstrate safety first. Setting the table is part of the anticipation of the event of mealtime. It is a great way to involve your child. It can be an enjoyable time with music or singing—something to get the child seeing the anticipation as opposed to the chore.

Talk to your child. With a positive attitude, you can actually improve the efficiency in the kitchen with the all the help from your child or children. Everyone should feel as if they are part of the family team. And the best teams function with equal participation. The kitchen used to be a place central to the relationship between a mom and her children. Doing homework and talking about school and friends while Mom made snacks and made dinner. Today, kitchens are showplaces with granite countertops and fancy appliances some of which are hardly used. Yes, parents are busy. But we have to start somewhere. We have to start being in the kitchen and using it, and sharing in it. Even if all you can do is one dinner a week in the kitchen, it can still become a time where memories are made. Conversation in the kitchen can lead to conversation at the table. Encourage and allow the conversation to evolve from the kitchen to family mealtime.

Tips/Summary

1. Involve your child in meal preparation.
2. Use a positive tone to imply privilege instead of doing a chore.
3. Choose age-appropriate tasks such as stirring, pouring and measuring.
4. Teach your teenager how to make basic dishes.
5. Have your child set the table.
6. Have conversations in the kitchen and during meal preparation.

SECRET #11

Set Appropriate Boundaries

It is most important at this stage in the game to set some appropriate boundaries. These boundaries will help continue the importance of healthy eating by continually affirming the commitment and respect we have for the meal and our bodies. Some of these boundaries include having table manners, eating foods in a certain order, when to have dessert, how to talk about food and the importance of gratitude. Each one has its own place, and each one will take some time to encourage and put into place. Many will take constant reinforcement. Parenting is an ongoing process and repetition and reinforcement are part of the job description, even when we would rather not have to say something over and over again.

Good Manners

Manners are cool. They really are. They used to be important, and then we forgot about their importance. Table manners are one of the many things that separate us from the animals. Many of you might be thinking, "I don't have time or energy to consider manners for a child that won't eat healthy foods," and that is partly true. Table manners are certainly not a first or even second step. Table manners can only be introduced once the previous chapters have been put into place, but they cannot be forgotten altogether. Also, certain table manners are not really appropriate until the child understands the language you are using. For example, as soon as a child is able to say "please" and "thank you" you can introduce the politeness of using these words at the table. When your child has the understanding you can then encourage the following: eating with the *correct* utensil, educating your child on the difference between finger food and utensil food, how to avoid spitting food out of the mouth, how to use a napkin, how to ask to leave the table for a bathroom or other need, sitting in the chair and chewing with our mouths closed. The last two deserve some extra explanation as they relate to digestion.

Proper Posture

Sitting with our bottom "glued" to the chair is a more important table manner than most of us think. Often picky eaters will squirm or wiggle in their chair, and encouragement to sit correctly is important. Too much wiggling can disrupt the digestive process, and this may cause discomfort in the child. Discomfort in the digestion of a picky eater will only work against all the effort to get the child to eat better. It is also important to create postural stability for the wiggler. Sometimes a child will wiggle if their feet cannot touch a solid base or if they have to reach too far up to feel comfortable. Use a footstool to give the child solid footing and a special chair or cushion to make sure the table height is between the belly button and the chest. Make sure hips, knees and ankles are at ninety degrees.

Chewing Food Well

Chewing food well is also important and essential for healthy digestion. Food mixes with the enzymes in our saliva which begins the breakdown of carbohydrates. When food is eaten too quickly, there may not be enough enzyme activity. This may contribute to undigested food particles in a person's bowel movement, and/or it may mean some indigestion, or it may even contribute to food sensitivities. Chewing food well is something that children do not often understand without instruction. Food should be chewed 10-20 times depending on how big the bite of food. Also chewing with their mouth closed avoids too much air entering the digestive system that may contribute to gas, bloating or indigestion.

Positive Food Talk

Another important boundary is to encourage positive talk about food, and reinforce the avoidance of negative talk about food. For example, a picky eater may lash out as the vegetable comes to the table with a sentence such as, "Broccoli is gross!" An appropriate response is "Broccoli is good for us and helps us stay healthy and strong."

Often a picky eater will talk about food in terms of like and dislike. "I don't like onions." An appropriate response is "That's okay, one day you might like onions." Or "You still have to try it, so that one day you will be able to like them." Remember it is only with repetition that new habits develop.

If your child has a negative response after trying a food, you can say something like, "Good for you for trying, and how about next time saying 'I don't care for onions.'" You can also avoid some of the negative talk in advance by talking about the benefits of the food served before anyone at the table has a chance to make a negative comment. For example, you bring dinner to the table and say, "I made chicken with broccoli tonight. Did you know broccoli is a super food and helps our bodies fight illness and disease?" Dinner conversation serves many functions, such as bonding with your children and reinforcing healthy self-esteem, but do not overlook the opportunity to teach your children about healthy eating.

Limiting Dessert

When the focus of mealtime is healthy eating, then desserts have to have their appropriate spot. Many families serve dessert every night. Eating dessert every night is often on top of a lunch that contained a sugar treat, and possibly an afternoon snack that contained sugar. This is a lot of sugar. Sugar interferes with our healthy taste buds and our desire for healthy foods. And let's not forget, sugar may stimulate hyperactivity; a concept many are unwilling to accept, but holds a lot of truth if you put it to your own personal test. The body's ability to handle sugar is also limited. Sugar is not a staple and may suppress the immune system and interfere in the overall wellness of the body. How often your family eats dessert needs to be part of the nutritional value system you created earlier.

A set of rules regarding sugar helps you maintain the boundaries regarding sugar and desserts as opposed to fighting a never ending battle on a regular basis. For example, some of you may decide that dessert is something you will allow on the weekends, some of you may decide it is something reserved for company and special occasions. No matter what you decide, dessert should not be at the end of every meal. You can use this reasoning: we work during the week, and we work on our health as well. So during the work week, we will avoid desserts. And never use dessert to bribe your picky eater to eat the healthy food. Studies show that using dessert to bribe will only reinforce the attitude that healthy food is something to avoid as much as possible.[20]

This before That

Your picky eater may also be smart enough to eat the food they like first which only serves to curtail the hunger and give them the stamina to resist the uncomfortable food. If your child eats a good amount of chicken first and then has no interest in eating the broccoli or carrots, then encouraging children to eat "this before that" is the strategy for you. "This before that" is a great way to set some boundaries about what is eaten first, so that you can use the child's hunger to your advantage. If your child is hungry, then you have far more leverage than if they have eaten something. Serve the unwanted food (such as the vegetable) on the plate with nothing else on the plate. Tell your child that when he or she has finished the vegetable on his or her plate that you will put the other food on his or her plate.

This strategy may not work if your picky eater has shown he or she has the capacity to go without eating altogether. Here's what you can do: First, be aware, some children are smart enough to refuse eating dinner completely knowing they can make up eating at another time. Make sure you know the reasons why your child is refusing food altogether. Is he or she waiting to snack later, or holding out for breakfast? If this is the case, make sure breakfast is very healthy. Next, you can tell your child that you want him or her to eat. Make sure your child knows you are not refusing him or her food, and when they are ready to eat they can eat the resistant food. If needed, you can also take a step back beginning with the child's point of first resistance. For example, if your child does not want a vegetable on the plate, you can begin with allowing the food to be on the plate. Do this for three or more days. Then, over the next few days ask your child to pick up what is on his or her plate and smell the food. Work with positive food talk during this time. The next step is to touch the food to his or her tongue. The next step is to taste the food. Eventually your goal should be chewing and swallowing the bite of resistant food.

One Bite for Every Year

Some children are willing to take one bite of the resistant food, and stop there. But then progress stops there. You need to think about the next course of action. A strategy that can help is "one bite for every year." This means that, if your child is four years old, he or she has to take four bites of the food he or she does not like. Not one bite but four. If he or she is six years old, then he or she has to take six bites, not three. "You are six years old so you have to take six bites." This uses their age and maturity to help encourage appropriate portions. If not, you may consider one bite success and then your picky eater does not get the health benefits of a full serving.

An Attitude of Gratitude

Part of what is often missing at the table is gratitude. Meals are often seen as a means for quick calories and hitting pleasure centers with high levels of sugar and salt. We forget that each time we sit down to a meal we are supposed to be nourishing our body. There are so many places in the world where children live without nourishment on an ongoing basis. Every time we eat we should be grateful for the food in front of us and the nourishment it provides us. Many people say a prayer, called grace, as a way to take a moment before eating to be grateful. But you do not have to be religious to take a moment of gratitude before you eat. It could sound like this, "Let's acknowledge our gratitude for this meal and the hands that prepared it. We are grateful that we live in a country where healthy food and clean water is available to us daily when so many people around the world go without." If we are grateful on a regular basis, a gentler and more respectful tone is set right from the beginning.

All in all, the attitude and posturing we take at the table sends a big message to our children and their behavior. If we consistently ask for table manners and good choices, we set the bar high enough for our children to want to better themselves even at the table. A respectful and positive attitude, even table manners are not something we are born with. These are to be learned. You can ask something better of your children. You can ask something better of yourself.

Tips/Summary

1. Recognize the need for appropriate boundaries at the table.
2. Begin to teach your child about table manners such as saying please and thank you, eating with a utensil, sitting in the chair, and chewing with our mouths closed.
3. Teach your child to sit with his or her bottom to the chair since it affects the digestive system.
4. Encourage your child to chew properly to help with optimal digestion.
5. Talk about food in a positive manner.

6. Positively correct your child when he or she uses negative talk about food.
7. Regulate dessert by including a guideline that fits your nutritional value system.
8. Use strategy "this before that" when appropriate and needed.
9. Use strategy "one bite for every year" when needed.
10. Keep and cover uneaten food for later, if needed.
11. Say grace or include a moment of gratitude before eating.

SECRET #12

Be Your Child's Cheerleader

The most challenging aspect of being the parent of a picky eater is the constant frustration over the lack of cooperation from the picky eater. When you feel overtired and stressed, you may want to throw in the towel. But your child's success comes, in part, from your continued belief in your child and your constant willingness to hope for his or her success without giving up. If you give up on your child, how will he or she ever believe she can face the challenges of life? How will he or she work through relationship challenges when they are older?

Many parents fail to see that, just like every other action we want our children to take, the process of changing their eating habits will require lots of repetition. Yes, we have to tell them one hundred and fifty million times to pick up their rooms, so yes, we will have to tell them that many times to eat their vegetables. But your success comes when they eventually eat what is served.

Your job as a parent is continual; and while we may not like certain aspects of our job, we have to take the good with the bad. When you begin to see the positive effects of healthy eating such as improved focus, concentration, and temperament, you will begin to have a strong conviction in your child's eating. You will see how it improves their performance and their success, and you will believe even more strongly. Allow this success to carry you through during the difficult meals, especially when you are reminding them of the new rules time and time again, and when the "on vacation" eating that no one in the family wants to stop doing must end. Remember, if you give up, your child is sure to give up.

You will be blessed for your commitment to your child. Especially when you see how they begin to embrace healthy eating as a young adult. You will feel blessed when you see the benefits to their health in eating healthy. You will feel blessed when their healthy sense of self enhances their self esteem. When it spills over into other areas, you will feel like it has been worth it. And it is worth it!

SAMPLE MEAL PLANS AND GROCERY LISTS

The following meal plans and matching grocery lists are a helpful resource for you to have an actual plan to put into place. These meals offer a variety of fruits and vegetables that help you prepare meals rich in nutrients while offering flexibility to encourage better eating of healthy foods.

Basic Meal Plan I

	BREAKFAST	LUNCH	SNACK	DINNER
SUNDAY	Pancakes with blueberries and pure maple syrup, sausage, and orange juice	Peanut butter and fruit spread sandwich, carrot sticks on the side	Popcorn and apple slices	Pork chops, fried rice (with chopped pineapple, red bell pepper), and sliced raw zucchini
MONDAY	Granola with unsweetened almond milk, strawberries	Quesadilla with cheese, slice pear and carrots	Apple and peanut butter	Homemade cheese pizza, Salad of Romaine and shredded carrot
TUESDAY	Waffles, maple syrup Sliced banana	Tuna fish sandwich, carrots sticks, apples (or tuna in avocado)	Rice cereal and fruit	Shrimp, snow peas, chopped tomato with pasta. Salad of spinach and shredded carrot
WEDNESDAY	Rice cereal with blueberries, almond milk	Turkey sandwich, potato chips and peaches	Celery and peanut butter with raisins	Tacos (ground turkey, lettuce, tomato and cheese) and refried beans
THURSDAY	Granola with strawberries and almond milk	Grilled cheese sandwich, apples and carrots	Popcorn and banana	Chicken breast, mashed potatoes, broccoli and salad with Romaine
FRIDAY	Waffles, strawberries, maple syrup	Turkey sandwich, peaches, raisins	Celery with peanut butter	Roasted chicken, kale, and spaghetti squash with Romano cheese
SATURDAY	Smoothie: banana, almond milk, frozen berries	Egg salad sandwich, carrots, potato chips	Apple slices and yogurt	Macaroni and mozzarella, salad of Red leaf lettuce, tomatoes

Grocery List
Meal Plan 1

Dry or Canned Goods
Arrowhead Mills or Bob's Red Mill Pancake mix (eaten 1x) (Budget friendly: any whole grain)
Granola (eaten 2x)
Vans Waffles (eaten 2x) (Budget friendly: Whole Grain)
Rice cereal (eaten 2x)
Heartland bread or other wholesome brand (2 slices eaten 6x)
Food 4 Life rice tortilla (eaten 1x) (Budget Friendly: whole wheat)
Kettle brand potato chips (eaten 2x)
Refried beans (eaten 1x)
Non-GMO Popcorn (eaten 2x)
Rice (eaten 1x)
Gluten Free pizza crust (eaten 1x) (Budget friendly: whole wheat)
Gluten Free pasta (eaten 1x) (Budget friendly: whole wheat)
Gluten Free macaroni pasta (eaten 1x) (Budget friendly: whole wheat)
Tomato sauce (eaten 1x for pizza)

Fruit
Blueberries (eaten 2x)
Strawberries (eaten 3x)
Banana (eaten 3x)
Frozen berries (served 1x in smoothie)
Pear (eaten 2x)
Apples (eaten 7x)
Peaches (eaten 2x)
Raisins (eaten 2x)
Pineapple (eaten 1x in fried rice)
Orange juice (drink 1x)

Condiments
Pure maple syrup (served 3x)
Peanut butter (eaten 4x)
Fruit spread (eaten 1x)

Vegetables
Carrots (eaten 7x, twice shredded into salad)
Celery (eaten 2x)
Red bell pepper (eaten 1x in fried rice)
Zucchini (eaten 1x)
Romaine lettuce (eaten 2x as salad)
Spinach (eaten 1x as salad)
Kale (eaten 1x)
Red Leaf lettuce (eaten 1x as salad)
Shredded lettuce (eaten 1x in tacos)
Snow peas (eaten 1x)
Tomatoes (eaten 2x)
Potatoes (eaten 1x)
Broccoli (eaten 1x)
Spaghetti squash (eaten 1x)
Avocado (optional-eaten 1x with tuna)

Dairy
Blue Diamond unsweetened almond milk (drink 4x)
Eggs (eaten 1x as egg salad)
Organic plain yogurt (eaten 1x)
Organic Mozzarella cheese (eaten 3x)
Organic Colby cheese (eaten 3x)
Romano cheese (eaten 1x)

Meat, Poultry, Seafood
Applegate Farms sausage (eaten 2x) (Budget friendly: Simple Truth)
Canned Albacore tuna (eaten 1x)
Applegate Farms sliced turkey breast (eaten 1x) (Budget friendly: Simple Truth)
Ground turkey (eaten 2x)
Pork chops (eaten 1x)
Shrimp (eaten 1x)
Ground beef (eaten 1x in meatloaf)
Chicken breast (eaten 1x)
Whole Chicken (eaten 1x)

Basic Meal Plan II

	BREAKFAST	LUNCH	SNACK	DINNER
SUNDAY	Basic omelet with turkey sausage, orange juice	Turkey sandwich with apple slices	Yogurt and blueberries	Steak, baked potato and Caesar salad
MONDAY	Granola with almond milk, strawberries	Peanut butter and honey sandwich, sweet potato chips, apple	Celery and peanut butter with raisins	Turkey burgers, baked French fries and apple sauce
TUESDAY	Toast with peanut butter and honey, blueberries	Turkey sandwich, celery sticks, banana	Rice cereal (dry) with raisins	Stuffed baked potato with cheese, salad of greens, tomato and sliced avocado
WEDNESDAY	Rice cereal with blueberries	Ham sandwich, potato chips and apples	Apples and crackers	Tuna casserole: pasta, tuna, cream soup and frozen peas. Cook pasta and toss ingredients Mixed green salad
THURSDAY	Granola with strawberries and almond milk	Chicken Tacquitos, apple sauce	Trail mix yogurt	Pan fried tilapia, Basmati rice, broccoli, sliced mango
FRIDAY	Toast with peanut butter and honey, banana	Turkey sandwich, apple	Celery with peanut butter	Red beans, rice and shredded cheese. Salad of Romaine and shredded carrots
SATURDAY	Smoothie: banana, almond milk, frozen mango	Grilled cheese, apple and tortilla chips	Apples and crackers	Chicken breast, spinach salad with shredded carrot, and steamed corn

Laura Kopec

Grocery List
Meal Plan II

Dry or Canned Goods
Granola (eaten 2x)
Heartland bread or other wholesome brand (eaten 2 slices eaten 8x)
Rice cereal (eaten 2x)
Sweet potato chips (eaten 1x)
Kettle brand potato chips (eaten 1x)
Tortilla chips (eaten 1x)
Rice Crackers (eaten 2x)
Trail mix (eaten 1x)
Gluten Free pasta (eaten 1x) (Budget friendly: whole wheat)
Cream soup (eaten 1x)
Basmati rice (eaten 1x)
Red beans (eaten 1x)

Fruit
Orange juice (drink 1x)
Strawberries (eaten 2x)
Blueberries (eaten 3x)
Banana (eaten 3x)
Frozen mango (eaten 1x in smoothie)
Mango (slices eaten 1x)
Apple (eaten 7x)
Applesauce (eaten 2x)
Raisins (eaten 2x)

Condiments
Peanut butter (eaten 5x)
Raw honey (eaten 3x)

Vegetables
Celery sticks (eaten 3x)
Potato (eaten 2x)
Romaine lettuce (eaten 2x)
Spinach (eaten 1x)
Mixed greens (eaten 2x)
French fries (eaten 1x)
Tomatoes (eaten 1x)
Avocado (eaten 1x)
Frozen peas (eaten 1x)
Broccoli (eaten 1x)
Carrots (eaten 2x)
Non-GMO corn (eaten 1x)

Dairy
Eggs (eaten 1x)
Blue Diamond unsweetened almond milk (drink 3x)
Organic Colby cheese (eaten 2x in stuffed baked potato, red beans)
Organic Mozzarella cheese (eaten 2x)
Organic plain yogurt (eaten 2x)

Meat, Poultry, Seafood
Applegate Farms turkey sausage (eaten 1x)
Applegate Farms sliced turkey breast (eaten 3x) (Budget friendly: Simple Truth)
Applegate Farms sliced ham (eaten 1x) (Budget friendly: Simple Truth)
Chicken taquitos (eaten 1x)
Steak (eaten 1x)
Ground turkey or turkey burgers (eaten 1x)
Canned Albacore tuna (eaten 1x)
Tilapia (eaten 1x)
Chicken breast (eaten 1x)

Basic Meal Plan III

	BREAKFAST	LUNCH	SNACK	DINNER
SUNDAY	Pancakes, uncured bacon, orange juice	Cucumber sandwich with apple slices	Crackers and cheese with apples	Roasted chicken, roasted sweet potato wedges, salad of mixed greens
MONDAY	Granola with almond milk, strawberries	Grilled cheese sandwich, carrot sticks, apple	Apple and peanut butter	Spaghetti with tomato sauce, Caesar salad
TUESDAY	Turkey sausage, sliced apples	Peanut butter and jam sandwich, celery sticks, oranges	Trail mix and banana	Pan fried tilapia rice with diced tomatoes, kale salad
WEDNESDAY	Rice cereal with blueberries	Turkey sandwich, potato chips and peaches	Celery and peanut butter with raisins	Shrimp and grits, Carrot salad with raisins
THURSDAY	Granola with strawberries and almond milk	Tuna sandwich, celery sticks, apples	Popcorn and apples	Chicken noodle soup, salad of butter leaf and avocado
FRIDAY	Rice cereal with almond milk, blackberries	Turkey sandwich, apple	Trail mix and banana	Taco Salad and rice
SATURDAY	Smoothie: banana, almond milk, frozen pineapple	English muffin personal pizza, carrot sticks	Apple with peanut butter	Pasta with diced ham and peas, mixed green salad

Grocery List
Meal Plan III

Dry or Canned Goods
Arrowhead Mills or Bob's Red Mill Pancake mix (eaten 1x) (Budget friendly: any whole grain)
Granola (eaten 2x)
Rice cereal (eaten 2x)
Heartland bread or other wholesome brand (2 slices eaten 6x)
Kettle brand potato chips (eaten 1x)
Gluten free English muffin (eaten 1x) (Budget friendly: whole wheat)
Rice crackers (eaten 1x)
Trail Mix (eaten 2x)
Non-GMO popcorn (eaten 1x)
Gluten free spaghetti (eaten 1x) (Budget friendly: whole wheat)
Basmati rice (eaten 2x)
Non-GMO Grits (eaten 1x)
Chicken Noodle Soup (eaten 1x)
Gluten free pasta (eaten 1x) (Budget friendly: whole wheat)
Non-GMO Corn Chips or Taco Shell Bowl (eaten 1x for taco salad)

Fruit
Orange juice (drink 1x)
Strawberries (eaten 2x)
Apple (eaten 9x)
Blueberries (eaten 1x)
Blackberries (eaten 1x)
Banana (eaten 4x)
Frozen pineapple (eaten 1x in smoothie)
Oranges (eaten 1x)
Peaches (eaten 1x)
Raisins (eaten 2x)

Condiments
Peanut butter (eaten 4x)
Fruit spread (eaten 1x)
Tomato sauce (eaten 2x, once for pizza)

<u>Vegetables</u>
Cucumber (eaten 1x)
Carrots (eaten 3x)
Celery (eaten 3x)
Sweet potato (eaten 1x)
Mixed greens (eaten 2x)
Romaine lettuce (eaten 2x, once for taco salad)
Kale (eaten 1x)
Butter leaf lettuce (eaten 1x)
Tomatoes (eaten 2x)
Avocado (eaten 1x)
Peas (eaten 1x)

<u>Dairy</u>
Blue Diamond unsweetened almond milk (drink 4x)
Organic Mozzarella cheese (eaten 1x)
Organic Colby cheese (eaten 3x)

<u>Meat, Poultry, Seafood</u>
Uncured Bacon (eaten 1x)
Applegate Farms turkey sausage (eaten 1x)
Applegate Farms sliced turkey breast (eaten 2x) (Budget friendly: Simple Truth)
Canned Albacore tuna (eaten 1x)
Chicken breast (eaten 2x)
Tilapia (eaten 1x)
Shrimp (eaten 1x)
Diced ham (eaten 1x)
Ground beef (eaten 1x for taco salad)
Whole chicken (eaten 1x for baked/roasted chicken)

Basic Meal Plan IV

	BREAKFAST	LUNCH	SNACK	DINNER
SUNDAY	Pancakes and eggs, orange juice	Chef salad: Romaine lettuce, hardboiled egg, diced chicken, shredded carrot	Chips and salsa	Chicken breast with tomatoes and leeks, Romaine salad
MONDAY	Granola with almond milk, strawberries	PBJ sandwich, grapes, tapioca pudding	Apple and peanut butter	Tortellini with asparagus and bell peppers tossed in olive oil, spinach salad
TUESDAY	Blueberry muffin, yogurt	Chicken noodle soup, apple	Cheese and crackers	Pork loin, mashed potato, carrots and peas
WEDNESDAY	Granola with yogurt, blueberries	Ham and cheese sandwich, potato chips and apples	Celery and peanut butter with raisins	Hash browns and egg, salad of Romaine and diced cucumber and tomato
THURSDAY	Raisin bran, almond milk	Tuna sandwich, celery sticks, apples	Cucumber and yogurt	Turkey chili: Black beans, pinto beans, tomato canned, ground turkey, and onion. Salad of mixed greens
FRIDAY	Egg, toast and orange juice	Grilled cheese, tomato soup, carrots	Trail mix and banana	Pan fried shrimp, snow peas and red bell pepper, rice and mixed greens salad
SATURDAY	Smoothie: banana, almond milk, frozen blueberries	English muffin homemade pizza, carrot sticks	Peanut butter and crackers	Linguine and clam sauce (or plain butter), Caesar salad

Grocery List
Meal Plan IV

Dry or Canned Goods
Arrowhead Mills or Bob's Red Mill Pancake mix (eaten 1x) (Budget friendly: whole grain)
Granola (eaten 2x)
Raisin bran (eaten 1x)
Heartland bread or other wholesome brand (2 slices eaten 4x)
Kettle brand potato chips (eaten 1x)
Non-GMO corn chips (eaten1x)
Rice crackers (eaten 2x)
Trail mix (eaten 1x)
Black beans (eaten 1x)
Pinto beans (eaten 1x)
Basmati rice (eaten 1x)
Blueberry muffin (eaten 1x)
Gluten free English muffin (eaten 1x) (Budget friendly: whole wheat)
Tomato soup (eaten 1x)
Chicken noodle soup (eaten 1x)
Canned clams (optional)
Gluten free linguine (eaten 1x) (Budget friendly: whole wheat)
Gluten free tortellini (eaten 1x) (Budget friendly: whole wheat)
Canned diced tomatoes (eaten 1x in chili)

Fruit
Orange juice (drink 2x)
Strawberries (eaten 1x)
Blueberries (eaten 1x)
Banana (eaten 2x)
Frozen blueberries (eaten 1x in smoothie)
Grapes (eaten 1x)
Apple (eaten 4x)
Raisins (eaten 1x)

Condiments
Peanut butter (eaten 4x)
Fruit spread (eaten 1x)
Tomato sauce (eaten 1x for pizza)
Salsa (eaten 1x)
Olive oil (eaten 1x)

Vegetables
Romaine (eaten 4x)
Spinach (eaten 1x)
Mixed greens (eaten 2x)
Carrots (eaten 4x)
Celery (eaten 2x)
Cucumber (eaten 2x)
Tomato (eaten 3x)
Leeks (eaten 1x)
Asparagus (eaten 1x)
Bell Pepper (eaten 2x)
Potato (eaten 1x)
Peas (eaten 1x)
Snow peas (eaten 1x)
Onion (eaten 1x)
Hash browns (eaten 1x)

Dairy
Egg (eaten 3x, once hardboiled in salad)
Blue Diamond unsweetened almond milk (drink 3x)
Organic plain yogurt (eaten 3x)
Tapioca pudding (eaten 1x)
Organic Mozzarella cheese (eaten 1x)
Organic Colby cheese (eaten 3x)
Organic butter (eaten 1x)

Meat, Poultry, Seafood
Chicken breast (eaten 2x)
Applegate Farms sliced ham (eaten 1x) (Budget friendly: Kroger Simple Truth)
Canned Albacore tuna (eaten 1x)
Pork loin (eaten 1x)
Ground turkey (eaten 1x)
Shrimp (eaten 1x)

BIBLIOGRAPHY AND RESOURCES

American Academy of Child and Adolescent Psychiatry. (2011). Children and Role Models. *Facts for Families Pages*, 99. Retrieved September 13, 2014 from http://www.aacap. org/AACAP/Families_and_Youth/Facts_for_Families/ Facts_for_Families_Pages/Children_and_Role _Models_99.aspx

American Cancer Society. *American Cancer Society Guidelines on Nutrition and Physical Activity for Cancer Prevention.* Retrieved on September 2, 2014 from http://www.cancer.org/acs/groups/cid/documents/ webcontent/002577-pdf.pdf

Aubele, T. & Reynolds, S. (2011). Have You Fed Your Brain Today? *Psychology Today.* Retrieved on September 5, 2014 from http:// www.psychologytoday.com/blog/primeyourgraycells/201109/ have-you-fed-your-brain-today

Azar, B. (2000). How do parents matter? Let us count the ways. *Monitor,* 31 (7), 62. Retrieved September 13, 2014 from http://www.apa. org/monitor/julaug00/parents.aspx

Cherry, K. (2014). What is the Difference between Extrinsic and Intrinsic Motivation? Retrieved on September 12, 2014 from psychology.about.com/od/motivation/f/difference-between-extrinsic-and-intrinsic-motivation.htm

Contento, I. (2011). *Nutrition Education: Linking Research, Theory and Practice.* (2ND Ed). Massachusetts: Jones and Bartlett Publishers.

Cook, E. & Dunifon, R. (2014). Do Family Meals Really Make a Difference? *Parenting in Context.* Retrieved on September 2, 2014 from http://www.human.cornell.edu/pam/outreach/upload/Family-Mealtimes-2.pdf

Fuhrman, J. (2005). *Disease Proof Your Child: Feeding Kids Right.* New York: St. Martin's Griffin.

Klein, S. (2011). 8 Reasons to Make Time for Family Dinner. *CNN Living.* Retrieved on September 2, 2014 from http://www.cnn.com/2011/10/25/living/family-dinner-h/

Kopec, L. (2013). *Let's Get Real about Eating: A practical guide to nutrition and health.* Indiana: Balboa Press.

Leman, K. (1995). *Bringing Up Kids Without Tearing Them Down.* Tennessee: Thomas Nelson Publishers.

Levine, M. (2012). *Teach Your Children Well.* Tennessee: Harper Collins.

O'Connor, A. (2012). 70% of Students Gain Weight During College: Study. *News & Views.* Retrieved on November 9, 2014 from http://news.health.com/2012/09/26/college-gain-weight/

Purdue University Center for Families Promoting Family Meals Project. *Family Meals Spell S-U-C-C-E-S-S.* Retrieved on September 2, 2014 from http://www.cfs.purdue.edu/cff/documents/promoting_meals/spellsuccessfatsheet.pdf

Savage, J., Fisher, J., & Birch, L. (2007). Parental Influence on Eating Behavior: Conception to Adolescence. *Journal of Law and Medical Ethics*, 35 (1), 22-34. PMC2531152. doi:10.1111/j.1748-720x.2007.00111.x

ENDNOTES

[1]   Fuhrman, J. (2005). *Disease Proof Your Child: Feeding Kids Right.* New York: St. Martin's Griffin. p.xviii-xix

[2]   Ibid

[3]   American Cancer Society. *American Cancer Society Guidelines on Nutrition and Physical Activity for Cancer Prevention.* Retrieved on September 2, 2014 from http://www.cancer.org/acs/groups/cid/documents/webcontent/002577-pdf.pdf

[4]   Kopec, L. (2013). *Let's Get Real about Eating: A practical guide to nutrition and health.* Indiana: Balboa Press. p. 5

[5]   Ibid, p. 83

[6]   Azar, B. (2000). How do parents matter? Let us count the ways. *Monitor,* 31 (7), 62. Retrieved September 13, 2014 from http://www.apa.org/monitor/julaug00/parents.aspx

[7]   Aubele, T. & Reynolds, S. (2011). Have You Fed Your Brain Today? *Psychology Today.* Retrieved on September 5, 2014 from http://www.psychologytoday.com/blog/primeyourgraycells/201109/have-you-fed-your-brain-today

[8]   Levine, M. (2012). *Teach Your Children Well.* Tennessee: Harper Collins.p, 116-117.

9   Cook, E. & Dunifon, R. (2014). Do Family Meals Really Make a Difference? *Parenting in Context.* Retrieved on September 2, 2014 from http://www.human.cornell.edu/pam/outreach/upload/Family-Mealtimes-2.pdf

10 Purdue University Center for Families Promoting Family Meals Project. *Family Meals Spell S-U-C-C-E-S-S.* Retrieved on September 2, 2014 from http://www.cfs.purdue.edu/cff/documents/promoting_meals/spellsuccessfatsheet.pdf

11 Ibid

12 Klein, S. (2011). 8 Reasons to Make Time for Family Dinner. CNN Living. Retrieved on September 2, 2014 from http://www.cnn.com/2011/10/25/living/family-dinner-

13 Purdue University Center for Families Promoting Family Meals Project. *Family Meals Spell S-U-C-C-E-S-S.* Retrieved on September 2, 2014 from http://www.cfs.purdue.edu/cff/documents/promoting_meals/spellsuccessfatsheet.pdf

14 Azar, B. (2000). How do parents matter? Let us count the ways. *Monitor,* 31 (7), 62. Retrieved September 13, 2014 from http://www.apa.org/monitor/julaug00/parents.aspx

15 Savage, J., Fisher, J., & Birch, L. (2007). Parental Influence on Eating Behavior: Conception to Adolescence. *Journal of Law and Medical Ethics,* 35 (1), 22-34. PMC2531152. doi:10.1111/j.1748-720x.2007.00111.x

16 American Academy of Child and Adolescent Psychiatry. (2011). Children and Role Models. *Facts for Families Pages,* 99. Retrieved September 13, 2014 from http://www.aacap.org/AACAP/Families_and_Youth/Facts_for_Families/Facts_for_Families_Pages/Children_and_Role _Models_99.aspx

17 Ibid

18 Contento, I. (2011). *Nutrition Education: Linking Research, Theory and Practice.* (2ND Ed). Massachusetts: Jones and Bartlett Publishers.

19 O'Connor, A. (2012). 70% of Students Gain Weight During College: Study. *News & Views.* Retrieved on November 9, 2014 from http://news.health.com/2012/09/26/college-gain-weight/

20 Contento, I. (2011). *Nutrition Education: Linking Research, Theory and Practice.* (2ND Ed). Massachusetts: Jones and Bartlett Publishers.

ABOUT THE AUTHOR

Laura Kopec, NDT, MHNE, MA, CNC

Laura received a Doctorate in Traditional Naturopathy from Trinity School of Natural Health, a Master of Science in Health and Nutrition Education from Hawthorn University, a Master of Arts from the University of Arizona, and a Nutritional Counseling Certificate from Trinity School of Natural Health.

Laura runs a consulting practice based in the North Dallas area where she sees clients in person and by phone. She is available for speaking engagements and workshops/lectures. Her first book is titled *Let's Get Real About Eating: A practical guide to nutrition and health.* ISBN: 978-1-4525-7427-1. Laura lives in Plano, Texas with her husband and three children. For more information about Laura visit her website at www.laurakopec.com

My name is _____, and every day I take care of my body!

How many times I need to eat healthy!	My Super Healthy Food Choices!	Sunday	Monday	Tuesday	Wednesday	Thursday	Friday	Saturday
1 serving	Power Fruit							
1 serving	Supercool Fruit							
1 serving	Rockin' Veggies							
1 serving	Supercool Veggies							
1 serving	Powerpacked Veggies							
1 serving	Awesome Veggies							
1 serving	Power Protein (beans, chicken, eggs, fish, beef and more!)							
1 serving	Supersmart Protein							
1 serving	Powerful Protein							
1 serving	Supersmart whole grains							
1 serving	Way to go whole grains							
Bonus	Today I tried a new food!							